The Ultimate Lunch Sirtfood Diet Recipes

Don't miss these 50 delicious and healthy recipes to give your body everything it needs

Anne Patel

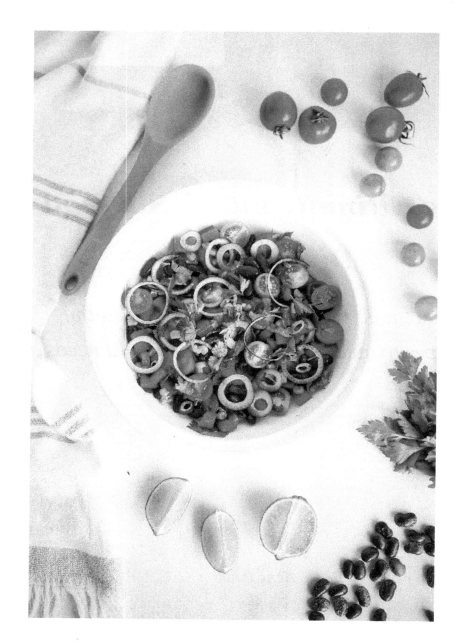

Table of Contents

Chapter 1: What is the Sirtfood diet

The Sirtfood Diet was created by Masters in Nutritional Medicine, Aiden Goggins and Glen Matten.

Their goal initially was to find a healthier way for people to eat, but people started losing weight quickly when they tested their program. With all the people in the world following diets hoping to lose pounds, they thought it would be selfish not to disclose their innovative health plan.

The plan they developed focuses on combining certain foods eaten in order to maximize the supply of nutrition to our body. There is an initial phase in which calories are limited to give the body a period to recover and eliminate accumulated waste. A maintenance phase follows this first phase to accustom the metabolism to the new foods you are ingesting. Throughout all stages, you will incorporate potent green juices and well-structured, well-planned meals.

The diet focuses on so-called 'sirtfoods,' plant-based foods that are known to stimulate a gene called sirtuin in the human body. Sirtuins belong to an entire protein family, called SIRT1 to SIRT7, and each has specific health-related connections. These proteins help separate and safeguard our cells from inflammation and other damage resulting from everyday activities, helping to reduce our risk of developing major diseases, particularly those related to aging.

Studies have shown that people live longer and healthier lives when they eat diets rich in these foods that activate sirtuin, free from diabetes, heart disease, and even dementia. So this diet was designed to restore a healthy body situation, and one of the byproducts of a healthy body is also the loss of excess weight.

The diet Sirtfood is neither a miracle cure nor a week-long program designed to quickly lose weight before beach holidays. If you are only interested in losing a few pounds and then returning to your old habits, there are certainly plans and diets that are more suited to your needs.

The Sirtfood diet is a project born to help you for the rest of your life, using delicious foods, but that will also improve your health. If you switch from a standard American diet (SAD) to a sirtfood diet, you will lose all the weight your body does not need.

A healthy body does not store extra energy. It asks for what it needs and uses it effectively.

The diet isn't designed to encourage you to starve or deprive yourself. The fact is, foods that are deficient in nutrients are designer made to deprive you and, though the calories are there in plenty, your cells are still starved for the nutrition to help you thrive. The Sirtfood Diet is the opposite of deprivation and starvation. It is nourishment and balance.

Most people following the SAD may use 20 ingredients in a month, let alone enjoy the sheer volume of choice ingredients from the 120 options you will learn about here.

In recent decades, an alarming number of people have come to the conclusion that healthy food is boring, and plants or, more specifically, vegetables are terrible tasting. This is because the foods we've become dependent on – packed with sugar, salt, and unhealthy fats – have chemically altered our connection to food. Our brains are essentially lying to us, and our taste buds have been compromised.

This is one of the reasons the week-long reset is so important. After this first week, you will be able to taste food differently. The more you expose yourself to the recommended plant-based foods, the more pleasure you get out of them.

Sirtuins are critical for our health, regulating many essential biological functions, including our metabolism, which, I'm sure you know, is very closely connected to our weight. It's also a key figure in determining our body composition, such as how much muscle we build and how much fat we retain.

Sirtuin genes regulate all this and more. They're also integral in the process of aging and disease.

If we can turn these genes on, we'll be able to protect our cells and enjoy better health for longer life. Eating sirtfoods is the most effective way to accomplish this goal.

Sirtfoods are all plant-based, and they have many more benefits, in addition to being sirtuin activators.

Our bodies require energy to operate, and the majority of this fuel comes from three primary macronutrients: carbohydrates, fats, and proteins. These macros largely control our metabolic system and regulate how the calories we consume get processed by our bodies. This is why most diets focus exclusively on micronutrition and require you to calculate calories.

Our bodies need more than just energy to survive than thriving, however, which is why micronutrients are so important. They don't impact our weight as obviously as macros, but they are our health foundations.

Micronutrients, such as vitamins, minerals, fiber, antioxidants, and phytonutrients, are supposed to be consumed along with our calories. Unfortunately, in the Standard American Diet (SAD), they're in very limited supply.

When your diet is primarily made up of large quantities of red meat and processed meats, pre-packaged foods, vegetable oils, refined grains and a lot of sugar, you will have an almost total lack of micronutrition.

Plant foods offer the most micronutrients per calorie consumed. Every edible plant has a unique nutritional profile, protecting you from an innumerable variety of illnesses.

Sirtfoods, and other plant-based sources of nutrition, give your body what it needs to stay young and disease-free, and, as a bonus, this will help you remain at an ideal weight.

The original Sirtfood Diet encourages you to commit to a one week reset phase and then a 2-week maintenance phase where you rely heavily on the Sirtfood green juice for a significant dose of nutrition along with meals rich in sirtfoods. Once the phases are complete, to retain your health for the rest of your life, you will need to continue incorporating these sirtfoods into your daily meals.

The Sirtfood Diet is not a miracle cure, but if you stick to these recipes, you'll not just impress your taste buds, but you'll also enhance nearly every aspect of your health. To get safe, you don't have to count calories or starve yourself, the youthful body you've always wanted.

Sirtfood Diet Phases

Every newbie needs to understand that the sirtfood diet does not start with a single list of ingredients in your hands. Its implementation and adaptation are more than mere selective grocery shopping. Every diet can only work effectively when we allow our body to embrace the sudden shift and change in food intake. Similarly, the sirtfood diet also comes with two phases of adaptation. If a dieter successfully goes through these phases, he can continue with the sirtfood diet easily. There are mainly two phases of this diet, which are then succeeded by a third phase in which you can decide how you want to continue the diet.

Phase One

The first seven days of this diet plan are characterized as Phase One. In this phase, a dieter must focus on calorie restriction and the intake of green juices. These seven days are crucial to initiate your weight loss and usually help to lose up to seven pounds if the diet is followed properly. If you find yourself achieving this target, that means that you are on the right track.

In the first three days of the first phase, a dieter must restrict this caloric intake to 1,000 calories only. While doing so, the dieter must also have green juice throughout the day, probably three times a day. Try to drink green juice per meal. The recipes given in the book are perfect for selecting from.

Many meal options can keep your caloric intake in checks, such as buckwheat noodles, seared tofu, some shrimp stir fry, or sirtfood omelet.

Once the first three days of this diet has passed, you can increase your caloric intake to 1,500 calories per day. In these next four days, you can reduce the green juices to two times per side. And pair the juices with more Sirtuin-rich food in every meal.

Phase Two

After the first week of the sirtfood diet, then starts phase two. This phase is more about the maintenance of the diet, as the first week enables the body to embrace the change and start working according to the new diet. This phase enables the body to continue working towards the weight loss objective slowly and steadily. Therefore, the duration of this phase is almost two weeks.

So how is this phase different from phase one? In this phase, there is no restriction on the caloric intake, as long as the food is rich in sirtuins and you are taking it three times a day, it is good to go. Instead of having the green juice two or three times a day, the dieter can have juice one time a day, and that will be enough to achieve steady weight loss. You can have the juice after any meal, in the morning or in the evening.

After the Diet Phase

With the end of phase two comes the time, which is most crucial, and that is the after-diet phase. If your weight loss target has not been reached by the end of step two, then you can restart the phases all over again. Or even when you have achieved the goals but still want to lose more weight, then you can again give it a try.

Instead of following phases one and two over and over again, you can also continue having good quality sirtfood meals in this after-diet phase. Simply continue the eating practices of phase two, have a diet rich in sirtuin and do have green juices whenever possible. The diet is mainly divided into two phases: the first lasts one week, and the other lasts 14 days.

The best 20 sirt foods

All these foods include high quantities of plant compounds called polyphenols, which can be thought to modify the sirtuin enzymes, therefore, excite their super-healthy added benefits.

Top 20 sirtfoods

1. Arugula (Rocket)
2. Buckwheat
3. Capers
4. Celery
5. Chilis
6. Cocoa
7. Coffee
8. Extra Virgin Olive Oil
9. Garlic
10. Green Tea (especially Matcha)
11. Kale
12. Medjool Dates
13. Parsley
14. Red Endive
15. Red Onions
16. Red Wine
17. Soy
18. Strawberries
19. Turmeric
20. Walnuts

What Is So Great About Sirtuins?

There are seven types of Sirtuins named from **SIRT1** to **SIRT7**. Although our understanding of the exact functions of all the Sirtuins is minimal, studies show that activating them can have the following benefits:

Switching on fat burning and protection from weight gain: Sirtuins do this by increasing the mitochondrion's functionality (which is involved in the production of energy) and sparking a change in your metabolism to break down more fat cells.

Improving Memory by protecting neurons from damage. Sirtuins also boost learning skills and memory through the enhancement of synaptic plasticity. Synaptic plasticity refers to synapses' capacity to weaken or strengthen with time due to decreased or increased activity. This is important because memories are represented by different interconnected networks of synapses in the brain, and synaptic plasticity is an important neurochemical foundation of memory and learning.

Slowing down the Ageing Process: Sirtuins act as cell guarding enzymes. Thus, they protect the cells and slow down their aging process.

Repairing cells: The Sirtuins repair cells damaged by re-activating cell functionality.

Protection against diabetes: this happens through prevention against insulin resistance. Sirtuins do this by controlling blood sugar levels because this diet calls for moderate consumption of carbohydrates. These foods cause increases in blood sugar levels; hence the need to release insulin, and as the blood sugar levels increase greatly, there is a need to produce more insulin.

Over time, cells become resistant to insulin, hence producing more insulin and leading to insulin resistance.

Fighting Cancers: The chemicals working as sirtuin activators affect the function of sirtuin in different cells, i.e. by switching it on when in normal cells and shutting it down in cancerous cells. This encourages the death of cancerous cells.

Fighting inflammation: Sirtuins have a powerful antioxidant effect that has the power to reduce oxidative stress. This has positive effects on heart health and cardiovascular protection.

Chapter 2: How do the Sirtfood Diet Works?

The basis of the sirtuin diet can be explained in simple terms or in complex ways. However, it's important to understand how and why it works so that you can appreciate the value of what you are doing. It is important to also know why these sirtuin rich foods help to help you maintain fidelity to your diet plan. Otherwise, you may throw something in your meal with less nutrition that would defeat the purpose of planning for one rich in sirtuins. Most importantly, this is not a dietary fad, and as you will see, there is much wisdom contained in how humans have used natural foods, even for medicinal purposes, over thousands of years.

To understand how the Sirtfood diet works and why these particular foods are necessary, we're going to look at their role in the human body.

Sirtuin activity was first researched in yeast, where a mutation caused an extension in the yeast's lifespan. Sirtuins were also shown to slow aging in laboratory mice, fruit flies, and nematodes. As research on Sirtuins proved to transfer to mammals, they were examined for their use in diet and slowing the aging process. The sirtuins in humans are different in typing, but they essentially work in the same ways and reasons.

The Sirtuin family is made up of seven "members." It is believed that sirtuins play a big role in regulating certain functions of cells, including proliferation, reproduction and growth of cells), apoptosis death of cells). They promote survival and resist stress to increase longevity.

They are also seen to block neurodegeneration loss or function of the nerve cells in the brain). They conduct their housekeeping functions by cleaning out toxic proteins and supporting the brain's ability to change and adapt to different conditions or to recuperate i.e., brain plasticity). They also help minimize chronic inflammation as part of this and decrease anything called oxidative stress. Oxidative stress is when there are so many free radicals present in the body that are cell-damaging, and by fighting them with antioxidants, the body can not keep up. These factors are related to age-related illness and weight as well, which again brings us back to a discussion of how they actually work.

You will see labels in Sirtuins that start with "SIR," which represents "Silence Information Regulator" genes. They do exactly that, silence or regulate, as part of their functions. Humans work with the seven sirtuins: SIRT1, SIRT2, SIRT3, SIRT4, SIRT 5, SIRT6 and SIRT7. Each of these types is responsible for different areas of protecting cells. They work by either stimulating or turning on certain gene expressions or by reducing and turning off other gene expressions. This essentially means that they can influence genes to do more or less of something, most of which they are already programmed to do.

Through enzyme reactions, each of the SIRT types affects different areas of cells responsible for the metabolic processes that help maintain life. This is also related to what organs and functions they will affect.

For example, the SIRT6 causes and expression of genes in humans that affect skeletal muscle, fat tissue, brain, and heart. SIRT 3 would cause an expression of genes that affect the kidneys, liver, brain and heart.

If we tie these concepts together, you can see that the Sirtuin proteins can change the expression of genes, and in the case of the Sirtfood diet, we care about how sirtuins can turn off those genes that are responsible for speeding up aging and for weight management.

The other aspect to this conversation of sirtuins is the function and the power of calorie restriction on the human body. Calorie restriction is simply eating fewer calories. This, coupled with exercise and reducing stress, is usually a combination for weight loss. Calorie restriction has also proven across much research in animals and humans to increase one's lifespan.

We can look further at the role of sirtuins with calorie restriction and using the SIRT3 protein, which has a role in metabolism and aging. Amongst all of the effects of the protein on gene expression, such as preventing cells from dying, reducing tumors from growing, etc.), we want to understand the effects of SIRT3 on weight for this book's purpose.

As we stated earlier, the SIRT3 has high expression in those metabolically active tissues, and its ability to express itself increases with caloric restriction, fasting, and exercise. On the contrary, it will express itself less when the body has high fat, high calorie-riddled diet.

The last few highlights of sirtuins are their role in regulating telomeres and reducing inflammation, which also helps with staving off disease and aging. Telomeres are sequences of proteins at the ends of chromosomes. When cells divide, these get shorter. As we age, they get shorter, and other stressors to the body also will contribute to this. Maintaining these longer telomeres is the key to slower aging. In addition, proper diet, along with exercise and other variables, can lengthen telomeres. SIRT6 is one of the sirtuins that, if activated, can help with DNA damage, inflammation and oxidative stress. SIRT1 also helps with inflammatory response cycles that are related to many age-related diseases.

Calories restriction can extend life to some degree. Since this and fasting are a stressor, these factors will stimulate the SIRT3 proteins to kick in and protect the body from the stressors and excess free radicals. Again, the telomere length is affected as well.

Having laid this all out before you, you should appreciate how and why these miraculous compounds work in your favor, keep you youthful, healthy, and lean If they are working hard for you, don't you feel that you should do something too?

50 Essential Lunch Recipes

1. Butternut pumpkin with buckwheat

Preparation Time: 5 Minutes

Cooking time: 50 Minutes

Servings: 4

Ingredients:

One spoonful of extra virgin olive oil, one red onion, finely chopped

One tablespoon fresh ginger, finely chopped

Three cloves of garlic, finely chopped

Two small chilies, finely chopped

One tablespoon cumin

One cinnamon stick

Two tablespoons turmeric

800g chopped canned tomatoes

300ml vegetable broth

100g dates, seeded and chopped

one 400g tin of chickpeas, drained

500g butter squash, peeled, seeded and cut into pieces

200g buckwheat

5g coriander, chopped

10g parsley, chopped

Directions:

Preheat the oven to 400 °.

In a frying pan, heat the olive oil and saute the onion, ginger, garlic, and Thai chili. After two minutes, add cumin, cinnamon, and turmeric and cook for another two minutes while stirring.

Add the tomatoes, dates, stock, and chickpeas, stir well and cook over low heat for 45 to 60 minutes. Add some water as required. In the meantime, mix the pumpkin pieces with olive oil. Bake in the oven for about 30 minutes until soft.

Cook the buckwheat according to the Directions and add the remaining turmeric. When everything is cooked, add the pumpkin to the other ingredients in the roaster and serve with the buckwheat. Sprinkle with coriander and parsley.

Nutrition:

Calories per serving 248.1 Total Fat .8.7g Saturated fat per serving 2.6g Monounsaturated fat per serving 1.5g Polyunsaturated fat per serving 4.0g Protein per serving 8.5g

2. Roasted Artichoke Hearts

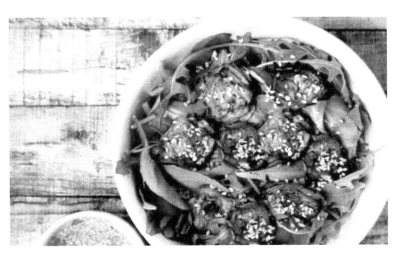

Preparation Time: 5 minutes

Cooking Time: 40 minutes

Servings: 3

Ingredients:

2 cans artichoke hearts

4 garlic cloves, quartered

2 tsp extra virgin olive oil

1 tsp dried oregano

salt and pepper, to taste

2-3 tbsp lemon juice, to serve

Directions:

Preheat oven to 375F.

Drain the artichoke hearts and rinse them very thoroughly.

Toss them in garlic, oregano, and olive oil.

Arrange the artichoke hearts in a baking dish and bake for about 45 minutes tossing a few times if desired.

Add salt and pepper to season and serve with lemon juice.

Nutrition:

Calories: 35 Fat: 20 g Carbohydrates: 3 g Protein: 1 g Fiber: 1 g

3. Beef Broth

Preparation Time: 5 minutes
Cooking Time: 40 minutes
Servings: 3

Ingredients:
4-5 pounds beef bones and few veal bones
1 pound of stew meat (chuck or flank steak) cut into 2-inch chunks
Olive oil
1-2 medium red onions, peeled and quartered
1-2 large carrots, cut into 1-2-inch segments
1 celery rib, cut into 1-inch segments
2-3 cloves of garlic, unpeeled
A handful of parsley stems and leaves
1-2 bay leaves
10 peppercorns

Directions:
Heat oven to 375F.

Rub olive oil over the stew meat pieces, carrots, and onions.

Put stew meat or beef scraps, stock bones, carrots, and onions in a large roasting pan.

Roast for approximately 45 minutes in the oven, turning everything halfway through the cooking.
Place everything from the oven in a large stockpot.

Pour some boiling water in the oven pan and scrape up all the browned bits and pour all in the stockpot.

Add parsley, celery, garlic, bay leaves, and peppercorns to the pot.

Fill the pot with cold water, over the top of the bones, to 1 inch.

Bring the stockpot to a regular simmer and then reduce the heat to low, so it just barely simmers. Cover the pan loosely and let it simmer for 3-4 hours, low and slow.

Scoop away the fat and any scum that rises to the surface occasionally.

After cooking, remove the bones and vegetables from the pot.

Strain the broth.

Let cool to room temperature and then put in the refrigerator.

The fat will solidify once the broth has chilled.

Discard the fat (or reuse it) and pour the broth into a jar and freeze it.

Nutrition:
Calories: 65 Fat: 1 g Carbohydrates: 2 g Protein: 3 g Fiber: 0 g

4. Salmon and Capers

Preparation Time: 5 minutes
Cooking Time: 40 minutes
Servings: 3

Ingredients:
75g (3oz) Greek yoghurt
4 salmon fillets, skin removed
4 tsp Dijon mustard
1 tbsp capers, chopped
2 tsp fresh parsley
Zest of 1 lemon

Directions:
In a bowl, mix the yoghurt, mustard, lemon zest, parsley, and capers.

Thoroughly coat the salmon in the mixture.

Place the salmon under a hot grill (broiler) and cook for 3-4 minutes on each side, or until the fish is cooked.

Serve with mashed potatoes and vegetables or a large green leafy salad.

Nutrition:
Calories: 283 Fat: 25 g Carbohydrates: 1 g Protein: 20 g Fiber: 0 g

5. Pasta Salad

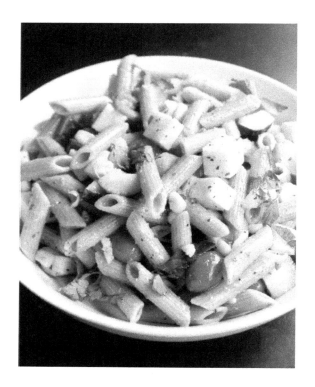

Preparation Time: 5 minutes
Cooking Time: 40 minutes
Servings: 3

Ingredients:
A plate of mixed greens ingredients
1 box (16 ounces) elbow pasta
4 cups of water
1 tbsp fit salt
2 tbsp olive oil
½ cup red onion, diced

1 cup simmered red peppers, daintily cut ¼ cup dark olives, cut

½ pound (8 ounces) crisp mozzarella, diced

½ cup slashed basil

Red wine vinaigrette ingredients

1 box (16 ounces) elbow pasta

4 cups of water

1 tbsp fit salt

2 tbsp olive oil

½ cup red onion, diced

1 cup simmered red peppers, daintily cut

¼ cup dark olives, cut

½ pound (8 ounces) crisp mozzarella, diced

½ cup slashed basil

Directions:

Amass pressure top, ensuring the weight discharge valve is in the seal position.

Select pressure and set it to high. Set time to 3 minutes.

Select start/stop to start.

Set up the red wine vinaigrette while the pasta is cooking.

In a blending bowl, join all vinaigrette fixings aside from olive oil.

Gradually speed in the olive oil until wholly joined.

Taste and alter seasonings as wanted.

Put in a safe spot.

At the point when weight cooking is finished, enable the strain to discharge for 10 minutes regularly.

Following 10 minutes, snappy discharge remaining weight by moving the weight discharge valve to the vent position.

Cautiously expel top when the unit has completed the process of discharging pressure.

Evacuate the pot and strain the pasta in a colander.

Move to a bowl and hurl with 2 tbsp of olive oil.

Spot bowl in cooler and enable pasta to cool for 20 minutes.

When pasta has cooled, mix in red onion, broiled peppers, dark olives, mozzarella, and basil.

Delicately crease in the red wine vinaigrette.

Serve quickly or cover and refrigerate for serving later.

Nutrition:
Calories: 248 Fat: 6 g Carbohydrates: 36 g Protein: 9 g Fiber: 0 g

6. Sirtfood Caramel Coated Catfish

Preparation time: 15 minutes

Cooking time: 45 minutes

Serving: 4

Ingredients:

1/3 cup water

2 tbsps. Fish sauce

2 shallots, chopped

4 cloves garlic, minced

1 1/2 tsps. Ground black pepper

1/4 tsp. red pepper flakes

1/3 cup water

1/3 cup white sugar

2 lbs. catfish fillets

1/2 tsp. white sugar

1 tbsp. fresh lime juice

1 green onion, thinly sliced

1/2 cup chopped cilantro

Directions:

Combine fish sauce and 1/3 cup of water in a small bowl; mix and put aside.

Combine together shallots, red pepper flakes, black pepper and garlic in another bowl and put aside.

Heat 1/3 cup of sugar and 1/3 cup of water in a big skillet placed over medium heat, stirring from time to time until sugar becomes deep golden brown. Stir in the fish sauce mixture gently and let the mixture boil. Mix and cook the shallot mixture.

Once the shallots have softened, add the catfish to the mixture.

Cook the catfish with cover for about 5 minutes each side until the fish can be easily flake using a fork. Transfer the catfish to a large plate, place a cover, and put aside. Adjust the heat to high and mix in a half tsp. of sugar.

Stir in any sauce that left on the plate and the lime juice.

Let it boil and simmer until the sauce has cooked down.

Drizzle the sauce on top of the catfish and sprinkle with cilantro and green onions.

Nutrition:
Calories per serving: 254 Carbohydrates: 4g Protein: 1g Fat: 0.5g
Sugar: 3g Sodium: 96mg Fiber: 1g

7. Lentil Tacos

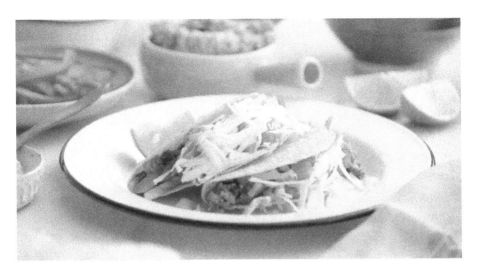

Preparation time: 10 minutes

Cooking time: 12 minutes

Servings: 8

Ingredients:

2 cups cooked lentils

½ cup chopped green bell pepper

½ cup chopped white onion

½ cup halved grape tomatoes

1 teaspoon minced garlic

½ teaspoon garlic powder

1 teaspoon red chili powder

½ teaspoon smoked paprika

½ teaspoon ground cumin

8 whole-grain tortillas

Directions:

Take a large skillet pan, place it over medium heat, add oil, and let it heat.

Add onion, bell pepper, and garlic, stir until mixed, and then cook for 5 minutes until vegetables begin to soften.

Add lentils and tomatoes, stir in all the spices and then continue cooking for 5 minutes until hot.

Assemble the tacos and for this, heat the tortillas until warmed and then fill each tortilla with ¼ cup of the cooked lentil mixture.

Serve straight away.

Nutrition:

Calories: 315 Fat: 7.8 g Protein: 13 g Carbs: 49.8 g Fiber: 16.2 g

8. Lentil and Quinoa Salad

Preparation time: 5 minutes

Cooking time: 15 minutes

Servings: 4

Ingredients:

2 medium green apples, cored, chopped

3 cups cooked quinoa

½ of a medium red onion, peeled, diced

3 cups cooked green lentils

1 large carrot, shredded

1 ½ teaspoon salt

1 teaspoon ground black pepper

2 tablespoons olive oil ¼ cup balsamic vinegar

Directions:

Take a large bowl, place all the ingredients in it and then stir until combined.

Let the salad chill in the refrigerator for 1 hour, divide it evenly among six bowls and then serve.

Nutrition:

Calories: 199 Fat: 10.7 g Protein: 8 g Carbs: 34.8 g Fiber: 5.9 g

9. Sloppy Joes

Preparation time: 5 minutes
Cooking time: 15 minutes
Servings: 4

Ingredients:

2 cups cooked lentils

2/3 cup diced white onion

1 medium sweet potato, peeled, chopped

1 medium red bell pepper, cored, diced

1 teaspoon minced garlic

¾ cup chopped mushrooms

1 teaspoon red chili powder

1 teaspoon paprika

1 teaspoon ground cumin

1 tablespoon brown sugar

1 tablespoon Worcestershire sauce

1 tablespoon olive oil ½ cup vegetable broth 15 ounces tomato sauce

Directions:

Take a large pan, place it over medium-high heat, add oil, and then let it heat.

Add onion, bell pepper, garlic, mushroom, and sweet potato, stir until mixed, and then cook for 8 minutes or more until potatoes turn tender.

Add lentils, stir in sugar and all the spices, pour in the tomato sauce and then cook for 3 minutes until thoroughly hot.

Pour in the broth, bring the mixture to a simmer, and then remove the pan from heat.

Ladle the sloppy Joes mixture over the bun and then serve.

Nutrition:

Calories: 125.3 Fat: 3.6 g Protein: 2.8 g Carbs: 20.1 g Fiber: 3 g

10. Lentil Burgers

Preparation time: 10 minutes

Cooking time: 10 minutes

Servings: 4

Ingredients:

2 cups cooked green lentils

2 tablespoons chopped white onion

4 ounces sliced mushrooms

1 teaspoon minced garlic

2 teaspoons garlic powder

2/3 teaspoon salt

½ teaspoon ground black pepper

1 tablespoon Worcestershire sauce

1 tablespoon yellow mustard

2 tablespoons olive oil

5 hamburger buns

Directions:

Place the cooked lentils in a blender, pulse until blended, and then tip the mixture into a medium bowl, set aside until required.

Place 1 tablespoon oil in a medium skillet pan, place it over medium heat, and when hot, add onion, mushrooms, and garlic.

Cook for 3 minutes, spoon the mixture to a food processor, add mustard, Worcestershire sauce, and 1 bun, and then pulse until slightly smooth.

Tip the mushroom mixture to lentil, and then stir until combined.

Add salt, black pepper, and garlic powder, stir until mixed, and then shape the mixture into four patties.

Over medium heat, place a skillet pan, add remaining oil and when hot, add patties and then cook for 3 minutes per side until golden brown.

Arrange the patty on a bun and then serve with favorite condiments.

Nutrition:
Calories: 184 Fat: 4 g Protein: 11 g Carbs: 28 g Fiber: 9 g

11. Potato Salad

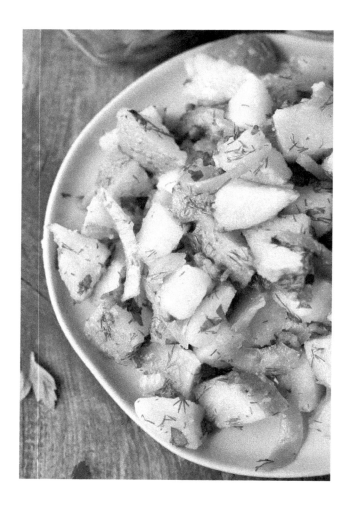

Preparation time: 5 minutes

Cooking time: 25 minutes

Servings: 4

Ingredients:

2 medium potatoes

2 medium tomatoes, diced

2 celery, diced

1 green onion, chopped

Directions:

Place a pan with the potatoes, cover with water, and then place the pan over medium-high heat.

Cook the potatoes for 20 minutes, and when done, drain them and let them cool.

Peel the potatoes, cut them into cubes, and then place them into a large bowl.

Add tomatoes, celery, and green onion, season with salt and black pepper, drizzle with oil and then toss until coated.

Divide the salad between three bowls and then serve.

Nutrition:

Calories: 268.5 Fat: 15.8 g Protein: 5 g Carbs: 21 g Fiber: 2.5 g

12. Ginger Brown Rice

Preparation time: 5 minutes
Cooking time: 40 minutes
Servings: 3

Ingredients:

1 cup brown rice, rinsed

1-inch grated ginger

½ of Serrano pepper, chopped

1 green onion, chopped

2 cups of water

Directions:

Take a medium pot, place it over medium-high heat, and then pour in water.

Add rice, green onion, Serrano pepper, and ginger, bring to a boil, switch heat to medium and then simmer for 30 minutes.

Divide rice among three bowls and then serve.

Nutrition:

Calories: 125 Fat: 1 g Protein: 3 g Carbs: 26 g Fiber: 0 g

13. Pasta with kale and Black Olive

Preparation time: 10 minutes
Cooking time: 40 minutes
Servings: 3

Ingredients:
60 g of buckwheat pasta
180 gr of pasta
Six leaves of washed curly kale
20 black olives
Two tablespoons of oil
½ chili pepper

Directions:
Cut the curly kale leaves into strips about 4 cm wide; cook them in salted boiling water for 5 minutes. Also, add the pasta to the pan. While the pasta is cooking, place the oil and olives in a non-stick pan. Drain the pasta and cabbage (keeping some cooking water aside) and add them to the olives. Mix well, adding, if needed, a little cooking water. Add the chili pepper and keep everything well.

Nutrition:
Calories per serving 372.7 Total Fat .28.0g Saturated fat per serving 2.7g Monounsaturated fat per serving 10.0g Polyunsaturated fat per serving 2.1g Protein per serving 3.6g

14. Asparagus Soup

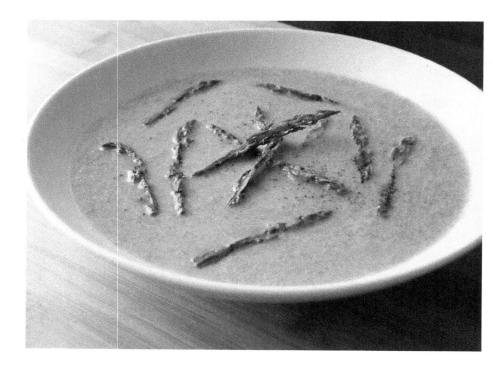

Preparation time: 5 minutes
Cooking time: 28 minutes
Servings: 6

Ingredients:
4 pounds potatoes, peeled, chopped
1 bunch of asparagus
15 ounces cooked cannellini beans
1 small white onion, peeled, diced
3 teaspoons minced garlic
1 teaspoon grated ginger
½ teaspoon salt

¼ teaspoon ground black pepper

1 lemon, juiced

1 tablespoon olive oil

8 cups vegetable broth

Directions:

Place oil in a large pot, place it over medium heat and let it heat until hot.

Add onion into the pot, stir in garlic and ginger and then cook for 5 minutes until onion turns tender.

Add potatoes, asparagus, and beans, pour in the broth, stir until mixed, and then bring the mixture to a boil.

Cook the potatoes for 20 minutes until tender, remove the pot from heat and then puree half of the soup until smooth.

Add salt, black pepper, and lemon juice, stir until mixed, ladle soup into bowls and then serve.

Nutrition:

Calories: 123.3 Fat: 4.4 g Protein: 4.7 g Carbs: 16.3 g Fiber: 4.1 g

15. Kale White Bean Pork chops

Preparation Time: 5 minutes
Cooking Time: 45 minutes
Servings: 4-6

Ingredients:
3 tbsp extra-virgin olive oil
3 tbsp chili powder
1 tbsp jalapeno hot sauce
2 pounds bone-in pork chops
Salt
4 stalks celery, chopped
1 large white onion, chopped
3 cloves garlic, chopped
2 cups chicken broth
2 cups diced tomatoes
2 cups cooked white beans
6 cups packed kale

Directions:
Preheat the broiler.
Whisk hot sauce, 1 tbsp olive oil and chili powder in a bowl.

Season the pork chops with ½ tsp salt.
Rub chops with the spice mixture on both sides and place them on a rack set over a baking sheet.

Set aside.

Heat 1 tbsp olive oil in a pot over medium heat.

Add the celery, garlic, onion, and the remaining 2 tbsp chili powder.

Cook until onions are translucent, stirring (approx. 8 minutes).

Nutrition:

Calories: 140 Fat: 6 g Carbohydrates: 14 g Protein: 7 g Fiber: 3 g

16. Tuna Salad

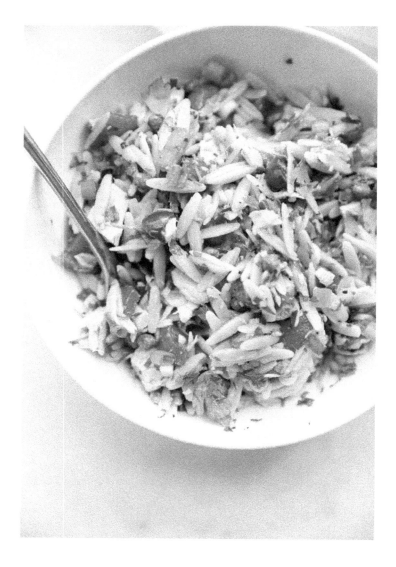

Preparation Time: 5 minutes

Cooking Time: 40 minutes

Servings: 3

Ingredients:

100g red chicory

150g tuna flakes in brine, drained

100g cucumber

25g rocket

6 kalamata olives, pitted

2 hard-boiled eggs, peeled and quartered

2 tomatoes, chopped

2 tbsp fresh parsley, chopped

1 red onion, chopped

1 celery stalk

1 tbsp capers

2 tbsp garlic vinaigrette

Directions:

Combine all ingredients in a bowl and serve.

Nutrition:

Calories: 240 Cal Fat:15 g Carbohydrates: 7 g Protein: 23 g

Fiber: 0 g

17. Turkey Curry

Preparation Time: 5 minutes

Cooking Time: 40 minutes

Servings: 3

Ingredients:

450g (1lb), turkey breasts, chopped

100g (3½ oz) fresh rocket (arugula) leaves

5 cloves garlic, chopped

3 tsp medium curry powder

2 tsp turmeric powder

2 tbsp fresh coriander (cilantro), finely chopped

2 bird's eye chilies, chopped

2 red onions, chopped

400ml (14fl oz) full-fat coconut milk

2 tbsp olive oil

Directions:

Heat the olive oil in a saucepan, add the chopped red onions and cook them for around 5 minutes or until soft.

Stir in the garlic and the turkey and cook it for 7-8 minutes.

Stir in the turmeric, chilies and curry powder then add the coconut milk and coriander cilantro).

Bring it to the boil, reduce the heat and simmer for around 10 minutes.

Scatter the rocket (arugula) onto plates and spoon the curry on top.

Serve alongside brown rice.

Nutrition:

Calories: 400 Fat:6 g Carbohydrates: 3 g Protein: 14 g Fiber: 0 g

18. Tofu and Curry

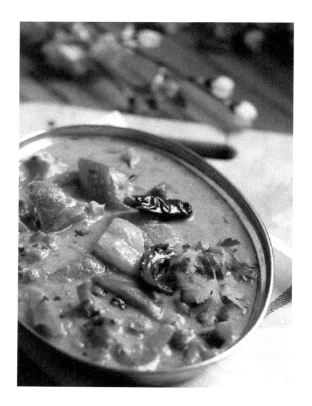

Preparation Time: 5 minutes
Cooking Time: 36 minutes
Servings: 4

Ingredients:
8 oz dried lentils (red preferably)
1 cup boiling water
1 cup frozen edamame (soy) beans
7 oz (½ of most packages) firm tofu, chopped into cubes

2 tomatoes, chopped

1 lime juices

5-6 kale leaves, stalks removed and torn

1 large onion, chopped

4 cloves garlic, peeled and grated

1 large chunk of ginger, grated

½ red chili pepper, deseeded (use less if too much)

½ tsp ground turmeric

¼ tsp cayenne pepper

1 tsp paprika

½ tsp ground cumin 1 tsp salt

1 tbsp olive oil

Directions:

Add the onion, sauté in the oil for few minutes then add the chili, garlic, and ginger for a bit longer until wilted but not burned.

Add the seasonings, then the lentils and stir

Nutrition:

Calories: 250 Fat:5 g Carbohydrates: 15 g Protein: 28 g Fiber: 1 g

19. Chicken and Bean Casserole

Preparation Time: 5 minutes

Cooking Time: 40 minutes

Servings: 3

Ingredients:

400g (14oz) chopped tomatoes

400g (14oz) tinned cannellini beans or haricot beans

8 chicken thighs, skin removed

2 carrots, peeled and finely chopped

2 red onions, chopped

4 sticks of celery

4 large mushrooms

2 red peppers (bell peppers), deseeded and chopped

1 clove of garlic

2 tbsp soy sauce

1 tbsp olive oil

1.75 liters (3 pints) chicken stock (broth)

Directions:

Heat the olive oil in a saucepan, put in garlic and onions and cook for 5 minutes.

Add in the chicken and cook for 5 minutes then add the carrots, cannellini beans, celery, red peppers (bell peppers) and mushrooms.

Pour in the stock (broth) soy sauce and tomatoes.

Bring it to the boil, reduce the heat and simmer for 45 minutes.

Serve with rice or new potatoes.

Nutrition:

Calories: 324 Fat: 11 g Carbohydrates: 27 g Protein: 28 g Fiber: 7 g

20. Prawn and Coconut Curry

Preparation Time: 5 minutes

Cooking Time: 35 minutes

Servings: 3

Ingredients:

400g (14oz) tinned chopped tomatoes

400g (14oz) large prawns (shrimps), shelled and raw

25g (1oz) fresh coriander (cilantro) chopped

3 red onions, finely chopped

3 cloves of garlic, crushed

2 bird's eye chilies

½ tsp ground coriander (cilantro)

½ tsp turmeric

400ml (14fl oz) coconut milk

1 tbsp olive oil

Juice of 1 lime

Directions:

Place the onions, garlic, tomatoes, chilies, lime juice, turmeric, ground coriander (cilantro), chilies and half of the fresh coriander (cilantro) into a blender and blitz until you have a smooth curry paste.

In a frying pan, heat the olive oil, add the paste and cook for 2 minutes.

Stir in the coconut milk and warm it thoroughly.

Add the prawns (shrimps) to the paste and cook them until they have turned pink and are thoroughly cooked.

Stir in the fresh coriander (cilantro).

Serve with rice.

Nutrition:

Calories: 163 Fat: 8 g Carbohydrates: 8 g Protein: 0 g Fiber: 1 g

21. Moroccan Chicken Casserole

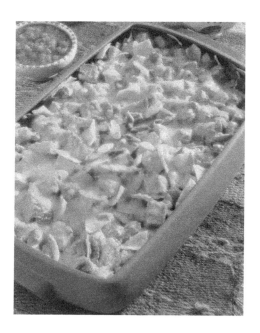

Preparation Time: 5 minutes

Cooking Time: 20 minutes

Servings: 3

Ingredients:

250g (9oz) tinned chickpeas (garbanzo beans) drained

4 chicken breasts, cubed

4 Medjool dates halved

6 dried apricots, halved

1 red onion, sliced

1 carrot, chopped

1 tsp ground cumin

1 tsp ground cinnamon

1 tsp ground turmeric

1 bird's eye chili, chopped

600ml (1 pint) chicken stock (broth)

25g (1oz) corn flour

60ml (2fl oz) water

2 tbsp fresh coriander

Directions:

Place the chicken, chickpeas (garbanzo beans), onion, carrot, chili, cumin, turmeric, cinnamon, and stock (broth) into a large saucepan.

Bring it to the boil, reduce the heat and simmer for 25 minutes.

Add in the dates and apricots and simmer for 10 minutes.

In a cup, mix the corn flour with the water until it becomes a smooth paste.

Pour the mixture into the saucepan and stir until it thickens.

Add in the coriander (cilantro) and mix well.

Nutrition:

Calories: 423 Fat: 12 g Carbohydrates: 0 g Protein: 39 g Fiber: 0 g

22. Chili con Carne

Preparation Time: 5 minutes

Cooking Time: 30 minutes

Servings: 3

Ingredients:

450g (1lb) lean minced beef

400g (14oz) chopped tomatoes

200g (7oz) red kidney beans

2 tbsp tomato purée

2 cloves of garlic, crushed

2 red onions, chopped

2 bird's eye chilies, finely chopped

1 red pepper (bell pepper), chopped

1 stick of celery, finely chopped

1 tbsp cumin

1 tbsp turmeric

1 tbsp cocoa powder

400ml (14 oz) beef stock (broth)

175ml (6fl oz) red wine

1 tbsp olive oil

Directions:

In a large saucepan, heat the oil, add the onion and cook for 5 minutes.

Add in the garlic, celery, chili, turmeric, and cumin and cook for 2 minutes before adding then meat then cook for another 5 minutes.

Pour in the stock (broth), red wine, tomatoes, tomato purée, red pepper (bell pepper), kidney beans and cocoa powder.

Nutrition:

Calories: 320 Fat: 21 g Carbohydrates: 8 g Protein: 24 g Fiber: 4 g

23. Tofu Thai Curry

Preparation Time: 5 minutes
Cooking Time: 30 minutes
Servings: 3

Ingredients:
400g (14oz) tofu, diced
200g (7oz) sugar snap peas
5cm (2-inch) chunk fresh ginger root, peeled and finely chopped 2 red onions, chopped
2 cloves of garlic, crushed
2 bird's eye chilies
2 tbsp tomato puree
1 stalk of lemongrass, inner stalks only
1 tbsp fresh coriander (cilantro), chopped
1 tsp cumin
300ml (½ pint) coconut milk
200ml (7fl oz) vegetable stock (broth)
1 tbsp virgin olive oil
juice of 1 lime

Directions:
In a frying pan, heat the oil, add the onion and cook for 4 minutes.
Add in the chilies, cumin, ginger, and garlic and cook for 2 minutes.

Add the tomato puree, lemongrass, sugar-snap peas, lime juice and tofu and cook for 2 minutes.

Pour in the stock (broth), coconut milk and coriander (cilantro) and simmer for 5 minutes.

Serve with brown rice or buckwheat and a handful of rockets (arugula) leaves on the side.

Nutrition:

Calories: 412 Fat: 30 g Carbohydrates: 27 g Protein: 14 g Fiber: 5 g

24. Roast Balsamic Vegetables

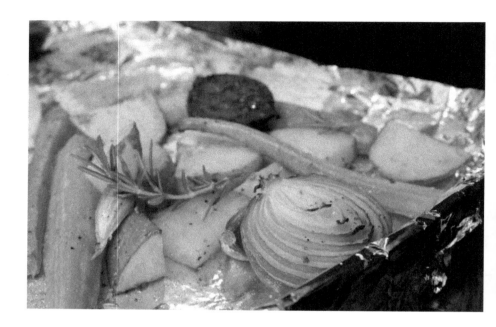

Ingredients:

4 tomatoes, chopped

2 red onions, chopped

3 sweet potatoes, peeled and chopped

100g (3½ oz) red chicory (or if unavailable, use yellow)

100g (3½ oz) kale, finely chopped

300g (11oz) potatoes, peeled and chopped

5 stalks of celery, chopped

1 bird's eye chili, deseeded and finely chopped

2 tbsp fresh parsley, chopped

2 tbsp fresh coriander (cilantro) chopped

3 tbsp olive oil

2 tbsp balsamic vinegar

1 tsp mustard

Sea salt

Freshly ground black pepper

Directions:

Place the olive oil, balsamic, mustard, parsley, and coriander (cilantro) into a bowl and mix well.

Toss all the remaining ingredients into the dressing and season with salt and pepper.

Transfer the vegetables to an ovenproof dish and cook in the oven at 200C/400F for 45 minutes.

Nutrition:

Calories: 70 Fat:0 g Carbohydrates: 8 g Protein: 2 g Fiber: 2 g

25. Chickpea Salad

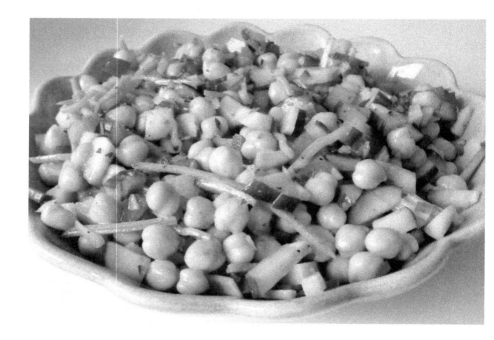

Preparation time: 5 minutes
Cooking time: 0 minutes
Servings: 2

Ingredients:

1 cup cooked chickpeas

16 leaves of butter lettuce

1 cup chopped zucchini

½ spring onion, chopped

1 cup chopped celery

1 cup grated carrot

1 tablespoon chopped cilantro

½ teaspoon salt

½ tablespoon lemon juice

Directions:

Take a large bowl, place all the ingredients in it, toss until mixed, and let it sit for 15 minutes.
Divide the lettuce leaves between two portions, top with the salad evenly and then serve.

Nutrition:

Calories: 166.6 Fat: 7.7 g Protein: 4.4 g Carbs: 20.8 g Fiber: 4.3 g

26. Vinaigrette

Preparation Time: 5 minutes
Cooking Time: 0 minutes
Servings: 1 cup

Ingredients:
4 teaspoons Mustard yellow
4 tablespoon White wine vinegar
1 teaspoon Honey
165 ml Olive oil

Directions:
1. In a bowl with a fork, whisk the mustard, vinegar, and honey until well combined.

2. Add the olive oil in small amounts while whisking with a whisk until the vinaigrette is thick.

3. Season with salt and pepper.

Nutrition: Calories: 45 Cal Fat: 0.67 g Carbs: 7.18 g Protein: 0.79 g Fiber: 0.8 g

27. Spicy Ras-El-Hanout Dressing

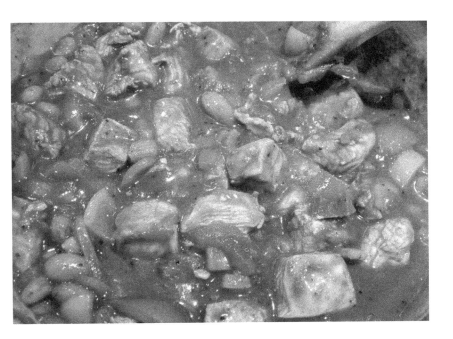

Preparation Time: 10 minutes

Cooking Time: 5 minutes

Servings: 1 cup

Ingredients:

125 ml Olive oil

1 piece Lemon (the juice)

2 teaspoons Honey

1 ½ teaspoons Ras el Hanout

½ pieces Red pepper

Directions:

1. Remove the seeds from the chili pepper.

2. Chop the chili pepper as finely as possible.

3. Place the pepper in a bowl with lemon juice, honey, and Ras-El-Hanout and whisk with a whisk.

4. Then add, drop by drop, the olive oil while continuing to whisk.

Nutrition: Calories: 81 Cal Fat: 0.86 g Carbs: 20.02 g Protein: 1.32 g Fiber: 0.9 g

28. Chicken Rolls With Pesto

Preparation Time: 15 minutes
Cooking Time: 20 minutes
Servings: 4

Ingredients:
2 tablespoon Pine nuts
25 g Yeast flakes
1 clove Garlic (chopped)
15 g fresh basil
85 ml Olive oil
2 pieces Chicken breast

Directions:
1. Preheat the oven to 175 ° C.

2. Bake the pine nuts in a dry pan over medium heat for 3 minutes until golden brown. Place on a plate and set aside.

3. Put the pine nuts, yeast flakes and garlic in a food processor and grind them finely.

4. Add the basil and oil and mix briefly until you get a pesto.

5. Season with salt and pepper.

6. Place each piece of chicken breast between 2 pieces of cling film

7. Beat with a saucepan or rolling pin until the chicken breast is about 0.6 cm thick.

8. Remove the cling film and spread the pesto on the chicken.

9. Roll up the chicken breasts and use cocktail skewers to hold them together.

10.Season with salt and pepper.

11. In a saucepan, melt the coconut oil and brown the chicken rolls over high heat on all sides.

12. In a baking dish, place the chicken rolls, place in the oven and bake for 15-20 minutes until they are done.
13.Slice the rolls diagonally and serve with the rest of the pesto.

Nutrition: Calories: 105 Cal Fat: 54.19 g Carbs: 6.53 g Protein: 127 g Fiber: 1.9 g

29. Vegetarian Curry From The Crock Pot

Preparation Time: 6 hours 10 minutes
Cooking Time: 6 hours
Servings: 2

Ingredients:

4 pieces Carrot

2 pieces Sweet potato

1 piece Onion

3 cloves Garlic

2 tablespoon Curry powder

1 teaspoon Ground caraway (ground)

¼ teaspoon Chili powder

1/4 TL Celtic sea salt

1 pinch Cinnamon

100 ml Vegetable broth

400 g Tomato cubes (can)

250 g Sweet peas

2 tablespoon Tapioca flour

Directions:

1. Roughly chop vegetables and potatoes and press garlic. Halve the sugar snap peas.

2. Put the carrots, sweet potatoes and onions in the slow cooker.

3. Mix tapioca flour with curry powder, cumin, chili powder, salt and cinnamon and sprinkle this mixture on the vegetables.

4. Pour the vegetable broth over it.

5. Cover the slow-cooker lid and let it simmer for 6 hours on a low setting.

6. Stir in the tomatoes and sugar snap peas for the last hour.

7. Cauliflower rice is a great addition to this dish.

Nutrition: Calories: 397 kcal Protein: 9.35 g Fat: 6.07 g Carbohydrates: 81.55 g

30. Fried Cauliflower Rice

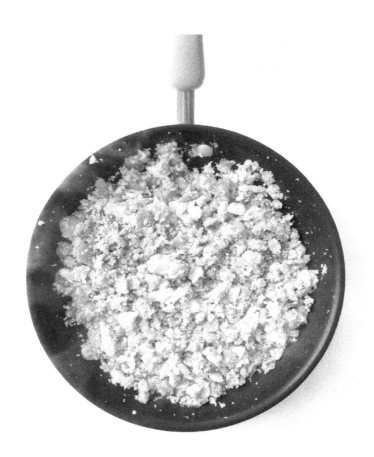

Preparation Time: 20 minutes

Cooking Time: 25 minutes

Servings: 4

Ingredients:

1 piece Cauliflower

2 tablespoon Coconut oil

1 piece Red onion

4 cloves Garlic

60 ml Vegetable broth cm fresh ginger

1 teaspoon Chili flakes

½ pieces Carrot

½ pieces Red bell pepper

½ pieces Lemon (the juice)

2 tablespoon Pumpkin seeds

2 tablespoon fresh coriander

Directions:

1. Cut the cauliflower into small rice grains in a food processor.

2. Finely chop the onion, garlic and ginger, cut the carrot into thin strips, dice the bell pepper and finely chop the herbs.

3. In a pan, melt 1 tablespoon of coconut oil and add half of the onion and garlic to the pan and fry briefly until translucent.

4. Add cauliflower rice and season with salt.

5. Pour in the broth and stir everything until it evaporates and the cauliflower rice is tender.

6. Remove the rice from the pan and set it aside.

7. Melt the rest of the coconut oil in the pan and add the remaining onions, garlic, ginger, carrots and peppers.

8. Fry until the vegetables are tender for a couple of minutes. Season them with a little salt.

9. Add the cauliflower rice again, heat the whole dish and add the lemon juice.

10.Garnish with pumpkin seeds and coriander before serving.

Nutrition: Calories: 261 Cal Fat: 35.61 g Carbs: 34.5 g Protein: 10.27 g Fiber: 8.4 g

31. Fried Chicken And Broccolini

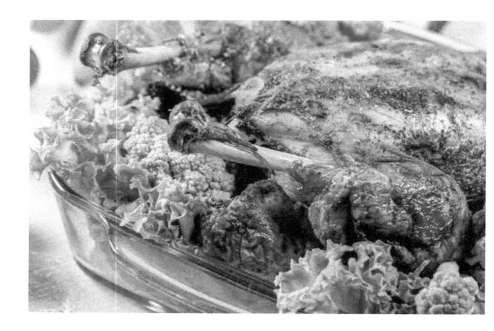

Preparation Time: 10 minutes

Cooking Time: 15 minutes

Servings: 5

Ingredients:

2 tablespoon Coconut oil

400 g Chicken breast

Bacon cubes 150 g

Broccolini 250 g

Directions:

1. Cut the chicken into cubes.

2. In a pan over medium heat, melt the coconut oil and brown the chicken with the bacon cubes and cook through.

3. Season with chili flakes, salt and pepper.

4. Add broccolini and fry.

5. Stack on a plate and enjoy!

Nutrition: Calories: 198 Cal Fat: 64.2 g Carbs: 0 g Protein: 83.4 g Fiber:0 g

32. Braised Leek With Pine Nuts

Preparation Time: 15 minutes

Cooking Time: 15 minutes

Servings: 4

Ingredients:

20 g Ghee

2 teaspoon Olive oil

2 pieces Leek

150 ml Vegetable broth

fresh parsley

1 tablespoon fresh oregano

1 tablespoon Pine nuts (roasted)

Directions:

1. Cut the leek into thin rings and finely chop the herbs. Roast the pine nuts in a dry pan over medium heat.

2. Melt the ghee together with the olive oil in a large pan.

3. Cook the leek until golden brown for 5 minutes, stirring constantly.

4. Add the vegetable broth and cook for another 10 minutes until the leek is tender.

5. Stir in the herbs and sprinkle the pine nuts on the dish just before serving.

Nutrition: Calories: 189 Cal Fat: 9.67 g Carbs: 25.21 g Protein: 2.7 g Fiber: 3.2 g

33. Sweet And Sour Pan With Cashew Nuts

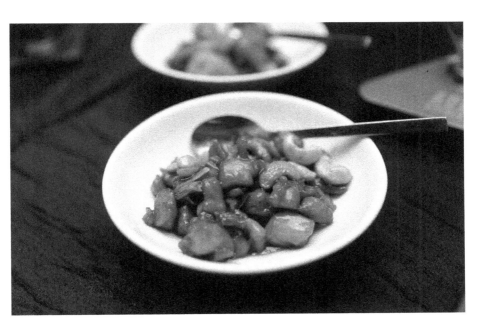

Preparation Time: 15 minutes

Cooking Time: 20 minutes

Servings: 4

Ingredients:

2 tablespoon Coconut oil

2 pieces Red onion

2 pieces yellow bell pepper

250 g White cabbage

150 g bok choi

50 g Mung bean sprouts

4 pieces Pineapple slices

50 g Cashew nuts

For the sweet and sour sauce:

60 ml Apple cider vinegar

4 tablespoon Coconut blossom sugar

1 ½ tablespoon Tomato paste

1 teaspoon Coconut-Aminos

2 teaspoon Arrowroot powder

75 ml Water

Directions:

1.Roughly cut the vegetables.

2. Mix the arrow root with five tablespoons of cold water into a paste.

3. Then mix in all the other ingredients for the sauce in a saucepan and add the arrowroot paste for binding.

4. Melt the coconut oil in a pan and fry the onion along with it.

5. Add the bell pepper, cabbage, bok choi and bean sprouts and stir-fry until the vegetables become a little softer.

6. Add the pineapple and cashew nuts and stir a few more times.

7. Pour a little sauce over the wok dish and serve.

Nutrition: Calories: 114 Cal Fat: 55.62 g Carbs: 55.3 g Protein: 30.49 g Fiber: 24.1 g

34. Butter Bean and Miso Dip with Celery Sticks and Oatcakes

Preparation Time: 5 Minutes

Cooking Time: 55 Minutes

Servings: 4

Ingredients:

2 x 14-ounce cans (400g each) of butter beans, drained and rinsed Three tablespoons extra virgin olive oil Two tablespoons brown miso paste

Juice and grated zest of

1/2 unwaxed lemon

Four medium scallions, trimmed and finely chopped One garlic clove, crushed

1/4 Thai chili, finely chopped celery sticks, to serve Oatcakes, to serve

Directions:

1. Simply mash the first seven ingredients together with a potato masher until you have a coarse mixture.

2. Serve with celery sticks and oat-cakes as a dip.

Nutrition: Calories 143. Total fat 3 g. Saturated fat Trace. Trans fat 0 g. Monounsaturated fat 2 g. Cholesterol Trace.

35. Spiced Scrambled Eggs

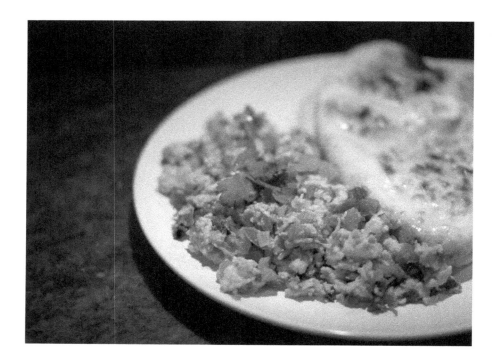

Preparation Time: 5 Minutes
Cooking Time: 15 Minutes
Servings: 4

Ingredients:
One teaspoon extra virgin olive oil
1/8 cup (20g) red onion, finely chopped 1/2 Thai chili, finely chopped Three medium eggs
1/4 cup (50ml) milk
One teaspoon ground turmeric
Two tablespoons (5g) parsley, finely chopped

Directions:

1. In a frying pan, heat the oil and cook the red onions and chili until soft but not browned.

2. Whisk together the eggs, milk, turmeric, and parsley.

3. Add to the hot pan and continue cooking over low to medium heat, continually moving the egg mixture around the pan to scramble it and stop it from sticking/burning.

4. When you have achieved your desired consistency, serve.

Nutrition: Calories 218.2. Total fat 15.3 g. Saturated fat Trace 6.3 g. Trans fat 0 g. Monounsaturated fat 5.5 g. Cholesterol Trace. 386.9 mg

36. Shitake Soup with Tofu

Preparation Time: 5 Minutes

Cooking Time: 15 Minutes

Servings: 4

Ingredients:

10g dried Wakame algae (instant)

1-liter vegetable stock

200g shitake mushrooms, sliced

120g miso paste

400g natural tofu, cut into cubes

Two spring onions

One red chili, chopped

Directions:

1. Bring the stock to boil, add the mushrooms, and cook for 2 minutes. In the meantime, dissolve the miso paste in a bowl with some warm stock, put it back into the pot together with the tofu, do not let it boil anymore.

2. Soak the Wakame as needed (on the packet), add the spring onions and Tai Chi, and stir again and serve.

Nutrition: Calories 137.4. Total fat 6.7 g. Saturated fat Trace 1.0 g. Trans fat 0 g. Monounsaturated fat 1.8 g. Cholesterol Trace. 0.0 mg

37. Chicken Curry with Potatoes And Kale

Preparation Time: 5 Minutes
Cooking Time: 45 Minutes
Servings: 4

Ingredients:

600g chicken breast, cut into pieces Four tablespoons of extra virgin olive oil

Three tablespoons turmeric Two red onions, sliced

Two red chilies, finely chopped

Three cloves of garlic, finely chopped

One tablespoon freshly chopped ginger

One tablespoon curry powder

One tin of small tomatoes (400ml)

500ml chicken broth

200ml coconut milk

Two pieces cardamom

One cinnamon stick

600g potatoes (mainly waxy)

10g parsley, chopped

175g kale, chopped

5g coriander, chopped

Directions:

1. Marinate the chicken in a teaspoon of olive oil and a tablespoon of turmeric for about 30 minutes. Then fry in a high frying pan at high heat for about 4 minutes. Remove from the pan and set aside.

2. In a pan with chili, garlic, onion, and ginger, heat a tablespoon of oil. Boil everything over medium heat and then add the curry powder and a

tablespoon of turmeric and cook, stirring regularly, for another two minutes. Add tomatoes, cook for another two minutes until finally chicken stock, coconut milk, cardamom, and cinnamon stick are added. Cook for about 45 to 60 minutes and add some broth if necessary.

3. In the meantime, preheat the oven to 425 °. Peel and chop the potatoes. Bring water to the boil, add the vegetables with turmeric, and cook for 5 minutes. Then pour off the water and let it evaporate for about 10 minutes. Spread olive oil with the potatoes on a baking tray and bake in the oven for 30 minutes.

4. When the potatoes and curry are almost ready, add the coriander, kale, and chicken and cook for five minutes until the chicken is hot.

5. Add parsley to the potatoes and serve with the chicken curry.

Nutrition: Calories 894 Carbs 162g Fat 22g Protein 25g Fiber 26g Net carbs 136g Sodium 2447mg Cholesterol 0mg

38. Buckwheat Noodles with Salmon And Rocket

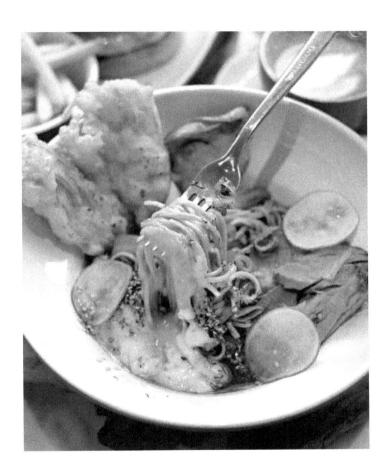

Preparation Time: 5 Minutes

Cooking Time: 45 Minutes

Servings: 4

Ingredients:

Two tablespoons of extra virgin olive oil One red onion, finely chopped

Two cloves of garlic, finely chopped

Two red chilies, finely chopped

150g cherry tomatoes halved

100ml white wine

300g buckwheat noodles

250g smoked salmon

Two tablespoons of capers

Juice of half a lemon

60g rocket salad

10g parsley, chopped

Directions:

1. In a coated pan, heat 1 teaspoon of the oil, add onions, garlic, and chili at medium temperature and fry briefly. Then add the tomatoes and the white wine to the pan and allow the wine to reduce.

2. Cook the pasta according to the directions.

3. Meanwhile, slice the salmon into strips, and when the pasta is ready, add it to the pan together with the capers, lemon juice, capers rocket, remaining olive oil, and parsley and mix.

Nutrition: Calories 320.1 Carbs. 25.2 Fat 13.0 g Protein 27.0 g

39. Caprese Skewers

Preparation Time: 5 minutes
Cooking Time: 30 minutes
Servings: 2

Ingredients:
4 oz. cucumber, cut in 8 pieces
8 cherry tomatoes
8 small balls of mozzarella or 4 oz. mozzarella cut in 8 pieces
1 tsp. of extra virgin olive oil
8 basil leaves
2 tsp. of balsamic vinegar
salt and pepper to taste

Directions:
1. Use 2 medium skewers per person or 4 small ones.

2. Alternate the ingredients in the following
order: tomato, mozzarella, basil, yellow pepper, cucumber and repeat.

3. Mix together the oil, vinegar, salt, and pepper and pour over the skewers
with the dressing.

**Nutrition: Calories: 280kcal, Fat: 8g, Carbohydrate: 14.g, Protein:
17g**

40. Baked Salmon with Stir Fried Vegetables

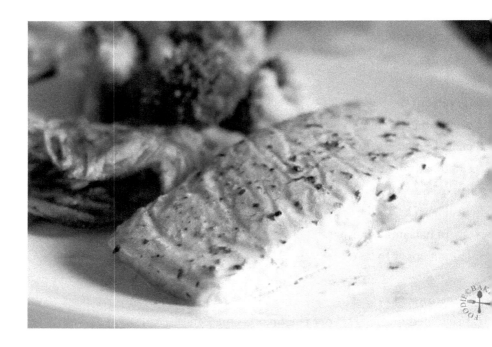

Preparation Time: 20 minutes

Cooking Time: 30 minutes

Servings: 2

Ingredients:

Grated zest and juice of 1 lemon

1 tsp. sesame oil

2 tsp. extra virgin olive oil

2 carrots cut into matchsticks

Bunch of kale, chopped

2 tsp. of root ginger, grated

8 oz. wild salmon fillets

Salt and pepper to taste

Directions:

1. Mix ginger lemon juice and zest together. In an oven proof dish, put the salmon and pour over the mixture of lemon ginger.

2. Cover with foil and leave for 30-60 minutes to marinate.

3. Bake the salmon at 375°F in the oven for 15 minutes.

4. While cooking heat up a wok or frying pan then add sesame oil and olive oil.

5. Attach the vegetables and cook for a few minutes, stirring constantly.

6. Once the salmon are cooked spoon some of the salmon marinade onto the vegetables and cook for a few more minutes.

7. Serve the vegetables onto a plate and top with salmon.

Nutrition: Calories 458kcal, Fat 13.2 g Carbohydrate 15.3 Protein 21.4g

41. Kale and Mushroom Frittata

Preparation Time: 15 minutes
Cooking Time: 30 minutes
Servings: 4

Ingredients:
8 eggs
½ cup unsweetened almond milk
Salt and ground black pepper, to taste
1 tbsp. extra virgin olive oil
1 red onion, chopped
1 garlic clove, minced
1 cup fresh mushrooms, chopped
1½ cups fresh kale, chopped

Directions:
1. Preheat oven to 350°F. In a large bowl, place the eggs, coconut milk, salt, and black pepper, and beat well. Set aside.

2. Heat the oil in a large ovenproof pan over medium heat and sauté the onion and garlic for about 3–4 minutes.

3. Add the kale salt, and black pepper, and cook for about 8–10 minutes.

4. Stir in the mushrooms and cook for about 3–4 minutes. Place the egg mixture on top evenly and cook for about 4 minutes, without stirring.

5. Transfer the pan in the oven and bake for about 12–15 minutes or until desired doneness.

6. Remove from the oven and leave to rest before serving for around 3-5 minutes.

Nutrition: Calories 151, Total Fat 10.2 g, Total Carbs 5.6 g, Protein 10.3 g

42. Trout with Roasted Vegetables

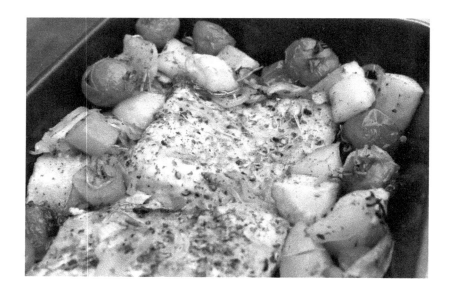

Preparation Time: 25 minutes

Cooking Time: 20 minutes

Servings: 2

Ingredients:

2 turnips, peeled and chopped

Extra virgin olive oil

Dried dill

1 lemon, juiced

2 carrots cut into sticks

2 parsnips, peeled and cut into wedges

2 tbsp. Tamari

2 trout fillets

Directions:

1. Put the sliced vegetables into a baking tray. Sprinkle with a dash of tamari and olive oil. Heat the oven to 400°F.

2. After 25 minutes, take the vegetables out of the oven and mix well.

3. Put the fish over it. Sprinkle with the dill and lemon juice. Cover with foil, and go back to the oven.

4. Turn down the oven to 375°F and cook till the fish is cooked through for 20 minutes.

Nutrition: Calories 154.0 Total Fat 2.2 g Carbohydrate 14.5 Protein 23.6

43. Mince Stuffed Peppers

Preparation Time: 15 minutes
Cooking Time: 60 minutes
Servings: 4

Ingredients:

4 oz. lean mince

¼ cup brown rice, cooked

2 large yellow

2 red bell peppers

1 tbsp. parmesan

2 tbsp. breadcrumbs

3 oz. mozzarella

1 egg

¼ cup walnuts, chopped

Salt and pepper, to taste

2 cups Arugula

2 tsp. extra virgin olive oil

Few drops Lemon juice

Cooking spray

Directions:

1. Preheat oven to 350° F.

2. In a bowl mix mince, parmesan, brown rice, egg and mozzarella. Mix well and set aside.

3. Cut peppers lengthwise, remove the seeds, fill them with the mince mix and put them on a baking tray.

4. Distribute breadcrumbs on top and lightly spray with cooking spray to have a crunchy top without adding calories to the recipe.

5. Cook for 50-60 minutes until peppers are soft. Let cool for a few minutes.
6. Serve stuffed peppers with an arugula salad dressed with olive oil, salt and a few drop of lemon.

Nutrition: Calories 375.1 Fat 8.2g Carbohydrate 24.7g Protein 15.3g

44. Vanilla Parfait with Berries

Preparation Time: 5 minutes
Cooking Time: 0 minutes
Servings: 1

Ingredients:

4 oz. Greek yogurt

1 tsp honey or maple syrup

1 cup mixed berries, frozen is perfect

1 tbsp. buckwheat granola

½ tsp Vanilla extract

Directions:

1. Mix yoghurt, vanilla extract and honey. Alternate yogurt and berries in a jar and top with granola.

2. Frozen berries are perfect if the parfait is made in advance because they release their juices in the yoghurt.

3. As far as granola, you can use a tablespoon of the one on page 88.

Nutrition: Calories: 318, Fat: 5.4g, Carbohydrate: 22.8g, Protein: 21.9g

45. Arugula Salad with Turkey and Italian Dressing

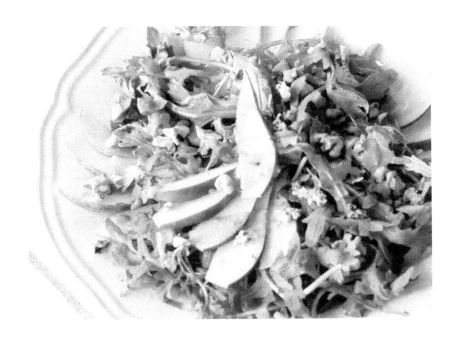

Preparation Time: 5 minutes

Cooking Time: 30 minutes

Servings: 2

Ingredients:

8oz. turkey breast

1 cup arugula

1 cup lettuce

2 tsp. Dijon mustard

1 tbsp. cumin

1/2 cup celery, finely diced

2 tsp. oregano

1/4 cup scallions, sliced

2 tsp. extra virgin olive oil

Salt and pepper to taste

Directions:

1. Grill the turkey and shred it. Set aside.

2. Mix lettuce and arugula on a plate. Evenly distribute shredded turkey, celery and scallions.

3. Mix all the dressing ingredients: mustard, olive oil, lemon juice, oregano, salt and pepper in a small bowl and pour over the salad just before serving.

Nutrition: Calories: 165 kcal, Fat: 2.9g, Carbohydrate: 13.6g, Protein:26.1g

46. Creamy Mushroom Soup with Chicken

Preparation Time: 10 minutes
Cooking Time: 40 minutes
Servings: 3

Ingredients:
2 cups vegetable stock
8 oz. mixed mushrooms, sliced
1 red onion, finely diced
1 carrot, finely diced
1 stick celery, finely diced
4 oz. chicken breast, cubed
1 tbsp. extra virgin olive oil
3 leaves sage

Directions:
1. Put 1 tbsp. oil in a skillet and cook chicken until lightly brown. Set aside.

2. Put the mushrooms in a hot pan with 1 tbsp. oil, celery, carrot, onion and sage and cook for 3 to 5 minutes.

3. Add the stock and let it simmer for another 5 minutes, then using a hand blender, blend the soup until smooth.

4. Add the chicken and cook for another 8 to 10 minutes until creamy.

Nutrition: Calories 302.0 Fat 3.5 g Carbohydrate 16.3 Protein 15 g

47. Super Easy Scrambled Eggs and Cherry Tomatoes

Preparation Time: 2 minutes
Cooking Time: 2 minutes
Servings: 1

Ingredients:

2 Eggs

1 tbsp. Parmesan or other shredded cheese Salt and pepper

½ cup cherry tomatoes

Directions:

1. Put eggs and cheese with a pinch of salt and pepper in a jar. Microwave for 30 seconds, then quickly stir with a spoon.

2. Put back in the microwave for 60 seconds and they are a ready to eat with cherry tomatoes.

3. In case you don't own a microwave, cook the scrambled eggs in a skillet for 2 minutes, stirring continuously until done.

Nutrition: Calories: 278, Fat: 5.4g, Carbohydrate: 12.8g, Protein: 18.9g

48. Lemon Ginger Shrimp Salad

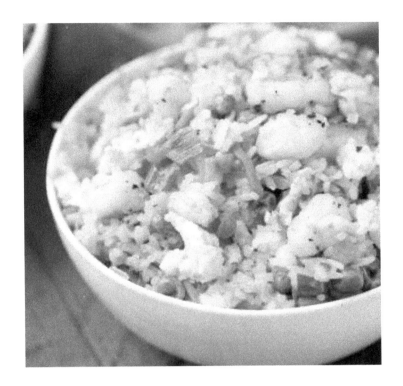

Preparation Time: 15 minutes

Cooking Time: 5 minutes

Servings: 2

Ingredients:

1 cup chicory leaves

½ cup arugula

½ cup baby spinach

2 tsp. of extra virgin olive oil

6 walnuts, chopped

1 avocado-peeled, stoned, and sliced

Juice of ½ lemon

8 oz. shrimps

1 pinch chili

Directions:

1. Mix chicory, baby spinach and arugula and put them on a large plate.

2. Heat a skillet on medium high temperature, put 1 tbsp. oil and cook shrimps with garlic, chili, salt and pepper until they are not transparent anymore (5 minutes)

3. Blend avocado with oil, lemon juice with a pinch of salt and pepper and distribute the dressing on top.

4. Chop the walnuts, put them on the plate as last ingredient and serve.

Nutrition: Calories: 353, Fat: 4.8g, Carbohydrate: 28.1g, Protein: 28.3g

49. Lemon Chicken Skewers with Peppers

Preparation Time: 5 minutes
Cooking Time: 15 minutes
Servings: 8

Ingredients:

8 oz. chicken breast

2 cups peppers, chopped

1 cup tomatoes, chopped

3 tsp. extra virgin olive oil

1 garlic clove

½ lemon, juiced

½ tsp paprika

½ tsp turmeric

1 handful parsley, chopped

Salt and pepper

Directions:

1. Cut the breast in small cubes and let it marinate with oil and spices for 30 minutes.

2. Prepare the skewers and set aside.

3. Heat a pan with oil. When hot add garlic and cook 5 minutes, the remove the clove.

4. Add peppers, tomatoes, salt and pepper and cook on high heat for 5-10 minutes.

5. Heat another pan to high heat, when very hot, put the skewers in and cook 10-12 minutes until golden on every side. Serve the skewers alongside the peppers.

Nutrition: Calories: 315 Fat: 20.9g Protein: 15.8g Carbohydrate: 5.4g

50. Overnight Oats with Strawberries and Chocolate

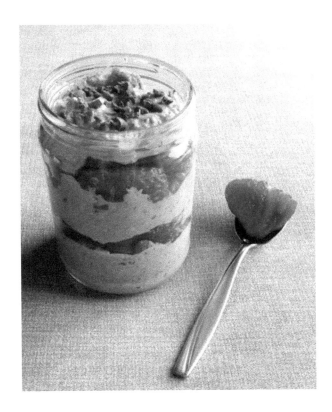

Preparation Time: 5 minutes + 8h

Cooking Time: 0 minutes

Servings: 2

Ingredients:

2 oz. rolled oats

4 oz. almond milk, unsweetened

2 tbsp. plain yoghurt

1 cup strawberries

1 tsp honey

1 square 85% chocolate

Directions:

1. Mix the oats and the milk in a jar and leave overnight. In the morning top the jar with yoghurt, honey, strawberries and chocolate cut in small pieces.

2. It can be prepared in advance and left in the fridge for up to 3 days.

Nutrition: Calories: 258, Fat: 3.3g, Carbohydrate: 29.8g, Protein: 13.6g

CPSIA information can be obtained
at www.ICGtesting.com
Printed in the USA
BVHW041055160321
602550BV00022B/1308